Always On Your Side Coaching

Progress Not Perfection

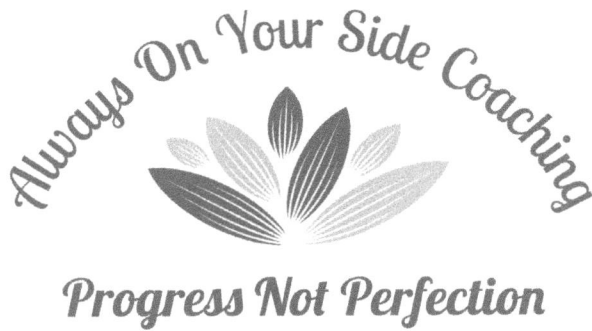

ALWAYS ON YOUR SIDE POWER OF 13

Your Common Sense Guide to Health and Wellness

I0096647

Paris Heinen

Published by Queen Publishing Agency
www.QueenPublishingAgency.com

ISBN 13 Softcover: 979-8-9886128-0-3
ISBN 13 Hardback: 979-8-9886128-1-0
ISBN 13 E-book: 979-8-9886128-2-7
ISBN 13 WORKBOOK: 979-8-9886128-3-4

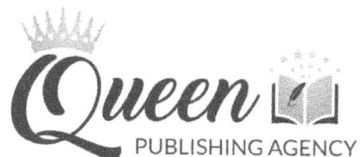
Queen PUBLISHING AGENCY

Dedicated to

My husband Don. Thank you for always supporting me and never saying my ideas are crazy. Your unconditional love and willingness to let me go for it every single time makes me love you more every day. Here's to another 35 years of crazy ideas.

My Parents. Fred and Glenadelle Downer for never saying, "Girl, that's impossible." Thank you for showing me hard work and kindness will get you everywhere. You taught me to see the good in people and do what I love.

My Girls, in no particular order. Vanessa, it all started with the belief that I could do this, and your agreement made me write this book. **Laura**, before I even thought about writing a book, you were telling me I needed a book AND a workbook and that I could do it. I don't know what I would do with you and your coaching. **Lena**, you are always there to bounce ideas off of and give me a truly honest opinion. **Sally and Marlene**, you both just trusted and had confidence when I said I wanted to start a coaching business; you jumped right in and said, of course, we will come work with you.

My Amazing Clients. Too many to name personally; I remember the night I said I was leaving Weight Watchers and starting my own coaching business. You all just trusted that it would work, and I knew what I was doing and came along for the ride. I learn something new from you all every time we meet. How blessed I am to have you all in my tribe.

=]Thank you from the bottom of my heart. Thank you for supporting me. Here's to an inspiring future.

~Coach Paris

Table of Contents

1.   Introduction
2.   Power of 13 #1 Cut portions in half on everything but vegetables
3.   Power of 13 #2 Move at least 30 minutes per day
4.   Power of 13 #3 Sleep at least 8 hours each night (non-negotiable)
5.   Power of 13 #4 Track your food and your feelings
6.   Power of 13 #5 Double your vegetable intake
7.   Power of 13 #6 Stretch "on purpose" 10 to 15 minutes every day
8.   Power of 13 #7 Read something positive 15 minutes every day
9.   Power of 13 #8 Learn about and incorporate healthy fats each day
10.   Power of 13 #9 Eat fruit, portion-controlled, each day
11.   Power of 13 #10 Create boundaries and enforce them
12.   Power of 13 # 11 Weight-bearing activity 15 to 30 minutes per day, 2 days a week
13.   Power of 13 #12 Limit White foods, sugar, salt, flour, rice, and pasta.
14.   Power of 13 #13 Pause and be mindful every day
15.   A few more things worth mentioning.
16.   What people are saying.
17.   Meet Coach Paris

Chapter 1

Always On Your Side Power of 13:
Your Common Sense Guide to Health and Wellness

~The Key to Living a Healthy Lifestyle is being
able to laugh along the way.
~Coach Paris

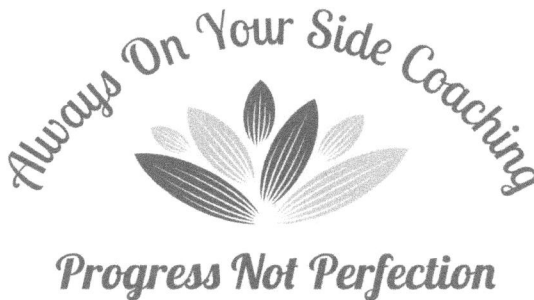

Always On Your Side Coaching

Progress Not Perfection

I remember lying on the laundry room floor, tears streaming down my face trying to button my jeans. Wondering how on earth I had let this happen. Back then, I had 55 pounds to lose and every excuse not to. I was busy with a new husband, two new stepkids, a full-time job, and, Oh yeah, no money. But I found a way to prioritize it, and my journey into health and wellness began. I found a program that worked for me: a support system and a voice to ensure everyone knew what I would need to succeed.

What are you waiting for? What will it take for you to prioritize your health and wellness? I have heard all the excuses anyone who wants to lose weight has. Reasons are just excuses holding you back from everything you want. Deciding to live a healthy lifestyle or lose weight should be an easy decision, but instead, we spend hours, days, and weeks coming up with excuses why we can't start now. Here are some I have heard and used myself.

- I will start after.....or on the 1st..... or on Monday.
- I am stressed (Or any emotion.)
- I don't have time (to prep, plan, exercise, focus, and make myself a priority)
- I have tried and failed before
- I will eat this now and burn it off later
- It's not fair that I have to eat healthy while everyone else can eat whatever they want
- I am too old
- I have too much to lose
- It takes too long
- Tracking is too time-consuming

There are hundreds more, but none that can not be challenged. If you want to lose weight and live a healthy lifestyle, you will make it your priority.

Let me enlighten you just a little bit. There is no "right time." You can always find a reason to wait. Are you waiting for someone else to do it for you? Me too! That's what I wanted. I wanted someone to spell it out, cook and exercise while I sat at home reading my book or watching TV. Guess what? No one is coming to the rescue. No one can do it for you. There is no magic pill. I can break it down into a straightforward, common-sense way of looking at your health and wellness. One that you don't have to be perfect at to be successful. It isn't about being skinny, it is about being healthy. Does this sound intriguing? Let me tell you a little bit about how the Power of 13 came to be.

I am Coach Paris. I have been a coach in the health and wellness industry for almost 24 years. I started my career in a Weight Watchers meeting room. I didn't know it then, but I was there to lose the weight I had gained back after losing it a few years before in the same Weight Watchers meeting room. My first experience with weight loss was after I had been married for a couple of years. We split everything, not in a good way like I do today. If I made a meatloaf, we split it. A big pot of pasta and sauce, we split it. My portions were out of control. I was cooking and eating way too much. So I found myself in a Weight Watchers meeting room at age 25, with 55 extra pounds to lose, and I followed the rules. I did it perfectly until I reached my goal, and then I didn't. I went back to my old way of eating and arrived back at my original weight and then some. Quick note: when you lose weight, you will have to continue doing what you did to lose it to keep it off. So here we are several years later, and I have to do it again! All 55 lbs. I followed the rules but had a very different outlook this time. I knew I would never want to do this again, so I learned and listened. I dug deep to understand my triggers and what worked for me. I took so much from the program, made it work for me, and kept my weight off for 24 years. When I reached my goal, I didn't run out the door and buy a quart of eggnog like I did the first time.

I applied for the job and became a Top Leader at Weight Watchers for 20 years. I loved my job and loved the company until I didn't. Like most of you, 2020 affected me. It affected us all in different ways, and I learned a lot about myself and what I wanted to do for the rest of my life. I spent the summer of 2020 studying and getting certified in 10 different areas of Life Coaching, including Health and Nutrition, Happiness, Goal Setting, Life Purpose, and so much more. I started to realize I wanted more and knew I could do it. Weight Watchers is one way, but there are many different ways to lose weight, and I wanted to allow people to find their right path. I quit my job on my 20th anniversary, and Always On Your Side Coaching opened two weeks later. I knew if I was going to start a health and wellness company, I would have to have guidelines. That is how the Always On Your Side Power of 13 came to be. I sat down at my dining room table with 20 years of Health and Wellness Coaching experience and started writing. There is no plan, just what you must do to live a healthy lifestyle. I wrote them down and then numbered them. 13 it was and is today. My clients often ask me why certain things didn't make the list (water, vitamins, dairy). It's because certain things are automatic and don't need space.

The Power of 13 is your common sense guide to Health and Wellness. It can be used with any diet plan you are doing, or it can stand alone. It is not 13 things you have to do every day; there are a few that when done daily, you will see more success. The Power of 13 is meant to help you feel successful every day, and trust me when I say you have done one or more already.

10.

Nothing in this book is rocket science. You will probably say "I know that" a lot while using it. It is meant to draw attention to the basics and make it easier to follow through. This book will walk you through the Power of 13 and give you tips and tricks to make each one a habit and understand what they mean. I will make it easy and fun. I encourage you to buy the workbook and use it with this book.

Here's to finding your right way to live a healthy life,

~Coach Paris

Be sure to sign up for updates and learn about our services on our website.

Alwaysonyoursidecoaching.com

We have Virtual 1:1 Coaching and Weekly Support groups available.

Coming 2024: We will have both online and in-person 12-week Always On Your Side Power of 13 Coaching courses.

Chapter 2

Power of 13

#1 Eat half portions of everything except vegetables

~Don't give up what you want most for
what you want in the moment.~
~Anonymous~

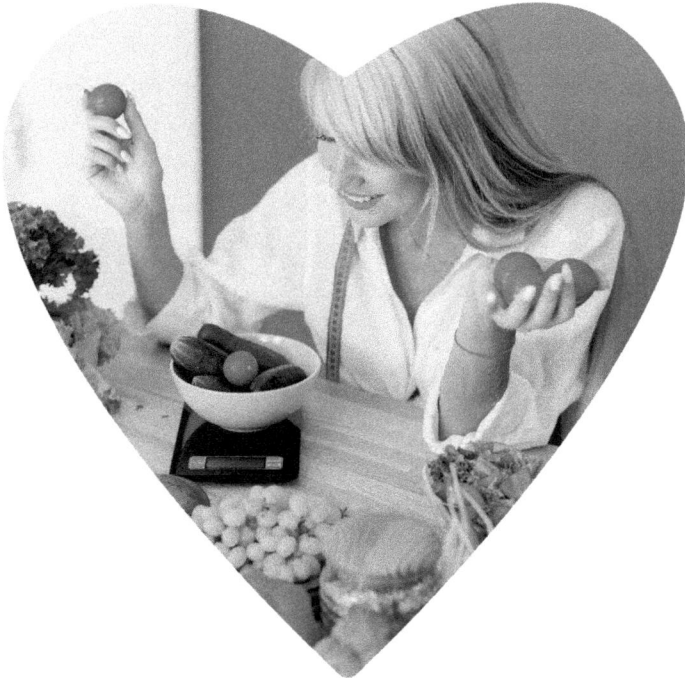

We live in a world of abundance and indulgence. We can not get enough of everything.

Our Portions have grown by 75% since the '70s. We started supersizing, and Big Gulps came into the picture. One of the biggest problems with that was it was usually cheaper to buy larger.

Nowadays, if you order one pizza, you will pay more than if you order pizza, breadsticks, and wings than if you just order one pizza. It's sad, and it can be confusing. Even looking at a nutrition label, we see the serving size and think that is what we must eat. You can eat ½ that portion and save calories.

Eating ½ portions can be an effective weight loss strategy because they help reduce overall calorie intake. When we eat less food, our bodies burn stored fat for energy, which can lead to weight loss over time. In addition, half portions can also help to regulate our hunger and satiety cues, allowing us to feel satisfied with less food and avoid overeating. By eating half portions, we can train our bodies to adjust to a lower calorie intake, which can lead to sustainable weight loss in the long term. Another benefit of eating smaller portions is that it can help to improve our digestion, reducing the risk of digestive problems such as bloating and indigestion. Overall, incorporating half portions into our diet can be a simple yet effective way to achieve and maintain a healthy weight while promoting good health and well-being.

#1 is all about cutting your portions to ½ on everything but vegetables. We will be doubling those soon. What is a Portion? This is important because you may be eating proper portions already, and we would not want you to cut those in half. But think about a few things: how often do you weigh and measure? Could you eat less and still feel satisfied? Have you tried?

14.

If you weighed out a 3-ounce chicken breast, I would not want you to cut that down to 1.5 ounces. It is time to start weighing and measuring. Here are some guidelines to get you started.

(remember you can eat more if you are still hungry BUT wait 15 minutes to see if it was enough.)

Healthy Choices and Portion Sizes

The key here is not guessing. You need to use measuring spoons or a scale. Below you will see a portion for a meal. Incorporating a healthy fat, protein, and vegetable/fruit at every meal

Main meal: I recommend you start with ½ your plate with non-starchy vegetables. You are filling the remainder with good-quality protein and a small starch.

Women:

Proteins: 3 to 4 ounces of chicken, turkey, lean beef, lamb, fish, seafood
½ to 1 cup of beans or legumes
1 cup skim or low-fat milk.
½ to 1 cup skim or low-fat yogurt. (no sugar added)
1/2 to 1-ounce Fat-free or low-fat cheese.
1 to 2 Eggs.
Starches: whole grain pasta, brown rice, grains ½ to ¾ cup cooked
Starchy vegetables (corn, potatoes, peas) ½ to ¾ cup
Salad Dressings and other condiments: 1 tablespoon
Crackers and chips: ½ the portion on the bag or box.
Nut Butters: 1 tablespoon
Fruit: 2 to 3 ½ cup portions
Nuts: ½ to 1 ounce

Men:

Proteins: 5 to 6 ounces of chicken, turkey, lean beef, lamb, fish, seafood
1 cup to 1.5 cups of beans or legumes
1 to 1.5 cups skim or low-fat milk.
1 to 1.5 cups skim or low-fat yogurt. (no sugar added)
1 to 2 ounces of fat-free or low-fat cheese.
2 to 3 eggs.
Starches: whole grain pasta, brown rice, grains 1 cup to 1.5 cups cooked
Starchy vegetables (corn, potatoes, peas) 1 cup to 1.5 cup
Salad Dressings and other condiments: 1 to 2 tablespoons
Crackers and chips the serving on the bag or box.
Nut Butters: 2 Tablespoons
Nuts: 1 to 2 ounces
Fruit 3 to 4½ cup portions

Simple ways to cut portions in half:

- Get familiar with what a portion is. Use a scale and measuring cups/ spoons consistently
- Cook less or if batch cooking, put extras away before you begin the meal
- Use smaller plates
- Drink 16 ozs. of water before the meal and drink water throughout the meal
- Put your fork down between bites and chew your food (slow down)
- Fill your ½ your plate with non-starchy vegetables
- The words "this is plenty" and "less is enough" are ways to reframe your thinking.

Use the Always On Your Side Power of 13 Workbook
to personalize your plan.

16.

Chapter 3

Power of 13

#2 Move your body for 30 minutes a day

~The more you move, the less you hurt~
~Coach Paris

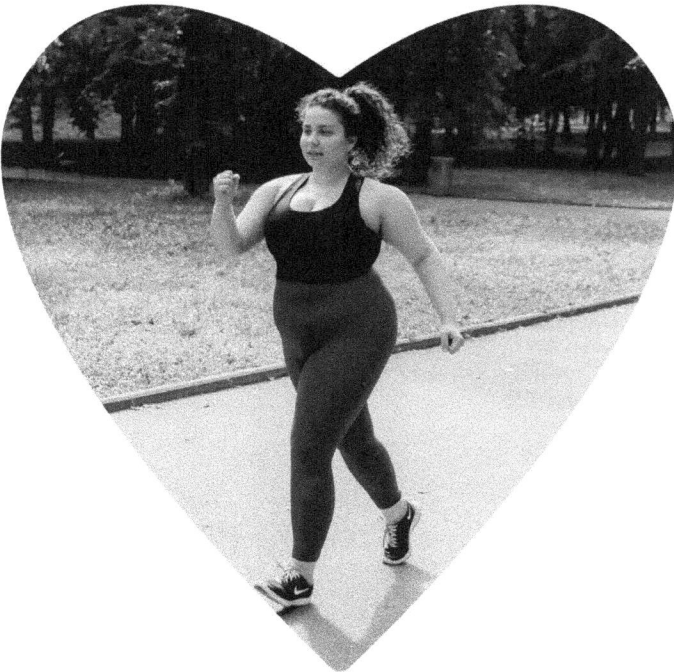

Moving your body with intention is one of the most important things you do for yourself every day. You have heard that sitting is the new smoking. The health risks of sitting all day are frightening. Challenging yourself to get up frequently can help with pain, mental clarity, and focus. When I am more active, I am less critical of my appearance. This is because I know I am doing the work.

Regular physical activity has been shown to have numerous health benefits, including reducing the risk of chronic diseases such as heart disease, diabetes, and cancer. It can also help to lower blood pressure, improve cholesterol levels, and strengthen bones and muscles. Physical activity is essential for maintaining a healthy weight and body composition. Regular exercise can help burn calories, increase metabolism, and improve body composition by reducing fat and muscle mass. Physical activity can positively impact mental health, reducing the risk of depression, anxiety, and other mental health issues. It can also improve cognitive function and reduce the risk of age-related cognitive decline. Physical activity can improve quality of life by increasing energy levels, reducing stress, and improving sleep quality. Overall, 30 minutes of daily activity is essential to a healthy lifestyle, providing numerous physical and mental health benefits.

The key to regular physical activity becoming a habit is finding what you enjoy doing. Exercise is one of the hardest things to "make yourself do." So finding something you look forward to will help you create a consistent schedule. In my practice, I have clients who would never miss a workout. They look at it as self-care and have it on their daily schedule. One of the hardest things about an activity is the start-stop start-stop that most of us do. When you do this, it is like starting over again and again. It is better to start slow and work up to something you can maintain. Begin by lowering your expectations. If you are not ready for 30 minutes, start with 5 minutes once a day and work up to 30 minutes.

18.

Also, studies show you don't have to do the 30 minutes consecutively. You can split it into 10 minutes 3 times a day or even 5 minutes 6 times daily. That takes away a lot of excuses about how you are too busy. Try new things. If you don't like them, keep searching. Also, there is a big difference between walking on a treadmill and walking outside. I am not a treadmill girl, but I will walk forever outside. I have friends who run and walk on treadmills and love it. They watch their shows, and it's convenient for them.

A Few Activity Suggestions and Benefits:

Walking is the top recommended cardio activity: whether inside or outside, you are less likely to hurt yourself (over running or jogging) are likely to hurt less or damage joints after a walk than a run. As you get stronger and build your endurance, you can speed up your time and work towards walking/jogging/running.

Cycling: Cycling improves strength, balance, and coordination. Indoor or outdoor cycling is a great way to build endurance and help you build muscle and lose weight.

Yoga: Yoga increases your balance and flexibility—two things you need to have as you age. Being steady on our feet and getting up and down off the floor is the key to independence as we age. Yoga keeps you strong and toned. You don't have to stand on your head to be good at yoga; learning just a few poses and doing them each day with consistency is enough to see all the benefits.

Pilates: Pilates promotes mobility and strength of all the major muscle groups in the body in a balanced fashion, focusing on the deep core muscles. It improves posture, flexibility, strength, balance, and body awareness.

Swimming/Aquacise: Aquacise was my form of exercise when I lost weight. I love how I feel in the water. I can do things I can't do on land. I continue to attend my classes twice a week. Swimming keeps your heart rate up but takes some of the impact stress off your body, building endurance, muscle strength, and cardiovascular fitness. It helps you maintain a healthy weight, healthy heart and lungs.

Aerobics: Aerobics classes have so many mental and physical benefits. Keep excess pounds at bay, Increase your stamina, Strengthen your heart, and boost your mood. Build your immunity and assist in weight loss and management.

Zumba/Dancing: Whether in a class or dancing all over the kitchen, dancing brings us joy. It's fun, easy, and uplifting. Turn up the music and just move. You know, dancing like nobody's watching. Zumba is the latest and greatest when it comes to classes. They are fun and great for your mental health. Find a class and try it out. It's a great way to tighten up and lose weight.

Strength training:

Much more important than we realize, strength training is an area that needs our focus weekly. 2 to 3 times a week. Increase Bone Density, Stabilize and Protect Joints, and

Reduce Body Fat. Strengthen your heart, Improve sleep quality, increase muscle size and strength, and support mental well-being.

Stop Overthinking it. If you don't have 30 minutes, do 5 or 10. Just get started.

These are all specific to exercise, but all movement counts. Remember yard work, house cleaning, anytime you are upright and moving. Just move. For those of you sitting at a desk daily, set a timer for 30 minutes, and when it goes off, get up and walk for 1 to 2 minutes. I set a timer and walked around the house. It gives me an extra 2500 to 3000 steps a day.

Bonus: I do not hurt nearly as badly when I move every 30 minutes.

Use the Always On Your Side Power of 13 Workbook to personalize your plan.

Chapter 4

Power of 13

#3 Sleep at least 8 hours a night (Non Negotiable)

~Sleep is the best form of meditation~
~Dalai Lama

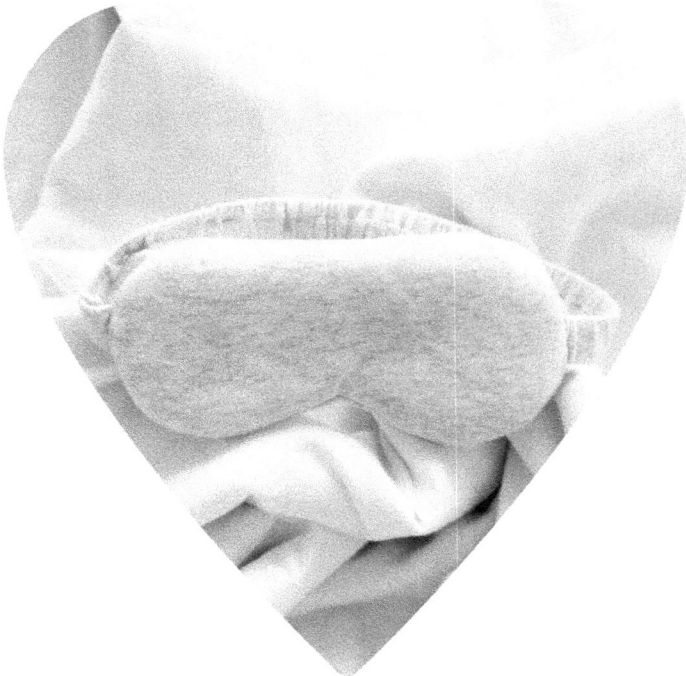

Remember when you were little, and someone told you when bedtime was—made you go to bed after brushing your teeth and a story? We hated that. 5 more minutes, one more book; I'm thirsty. Fast forward to today, and we still fight sleep; we don't have anyone making the rules, so we stay up a little later to finish a few more things. We struggle the next day, yawning, drinking too much coffee, and complaining we are tired. Sleep is vital to good health. Most of us do not take it seriously enough. Adults need 8 hours of quality sleep every single night.

Getting 8 hours of sleep is essential for several reasons. First, it allows our bodies to rest and recover from the physical and mental stresses of the day. During sleep, our bodies repair damaged tissues and cells, and our brains consolidate memories and process information. Do you feel like you need to remember things the way you used to?

Second, getting enough sleep helps to regulate our hormones, which can affect our mood, appetite, and metabolism. Lack of sleep has been linked to an increased risk of obesity, diabetes, and cardiovascular disease. Third, sleep is critical in maintaining a healthy immune system, which is important for fighting infections and diseases. Lastly, getting enough sleep is essential for mental and emotional well-being. Chronic sleep deprivation has been linked to an increased risk of depression, anxiety, and other mental health issues. Overall, getting 8 hours of sleep is important for our physical, mental, and emotional health and should be prioritized as part of a healthy lifestyle.

Non Negotiable: there are very few places I say this in health and wellness, but here I really mean it. Yes, you may think your 6 to 7 hours is getting the job done, but try 8, see how much better you feel, and function overall.

You need to create a sleep routine that you use every night. Remember the routine you had when you were little? Start 45 minutes to 1 hour before you need to be lights out. Repeated behaviors result in positive results.

24.

Create yours to match your lifestyle. Here are some ideas to get you started.

- Put away electronics—NO phones or computers in the bedroom. Yes, you read that right it is the hardest habit to break, but you can and must do it. No excuses. This is the #1 reason people are not sleeping. If you have to have your phone for emergencies, plug it in across the room from you.
- Decide on a set bedtime. The best thing you can do is go to bed at the same time every night and get up at the same time. Not always realistic, so be sure you are getting 8 hours by deciding what time you have to get up and be in bed asleep 8 hours before. (Need to be up at six lights out by 10)
- Wash your face and brush your teeth.
- Take a warm bath or shower. The temperature is really important. No hot or cold water (stay warm). Your body takes over an hour to regulate temperatures and will keep you up while doing it. So be careful with the temperature.
- Listen to music.
- Stretch, breathe, and relax. No heavy workouts, but stretching is so good for you.
- Practice meditation.
- Read a good book. (Reminder not on your phone)

Let's get you sleeping and see how quickly your health improves—mental clarity, less likely to make poor food choices, and easier to get active. Don't overlook this one. It is #3 for a reason. It is very important. You will lose more weight if you get better sleep!

Use the Always On Your Side Power of 13 Workbook
to personalize your plan.

Chapter 5

Power of 13

#4 Track food and feelings

~Knowledge is power; the more you know, the more you know~
~Coach Paris

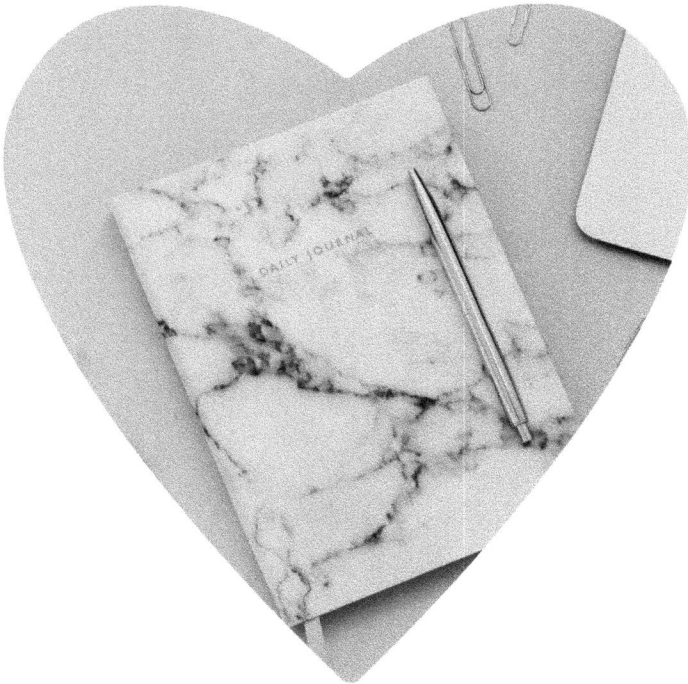

Every "diet" program out there says you need to track your food. If everyone says we need to do it, there must be something to it. Most people I talk to say they lose more weight when they track. However, knowing and doing is something completely different. It is also the 1st thing most people stop doing when they are trying to lose weight. The main reason we stop tracking is because we don't want to know. But we need to reframe why we are tracking.   Tracking your food gives you information. It shows you what you ate and helps you see what filled you up and sticks with you. Helping you understand the foods that fill you and keep you full is the key to a healthy lifestyle. When it comes to tracking your food, it gives you information on what works for you specifically.

Tracking your food intake can have several benefits for your health and well-being. First, it can help you become more aware of what you eat and how much. This can be especially helpful if you are trying to lose weight or make dietary changes. By tracking your food intake, you can identify areas where you may be consuming too many calories or not getting enough of certain nutrients. Second, tracking your food intake can help you set and achieve dietary goals. For example, you may set a goal to eat more fruits and vegetables or reduce your saturated fat intake. You can see how well you meet your goals and adjust as needed by tracking your progress. Third, it can help you identify patterns in your eating behavior, such as emotional eating or eating out of boredom. This can help you develop strategies for managing these behaviors and making healthier choices. Fourth, it can provide motivation and accountability. This can help you stay focused on your goals and make healthier choices throughout the day. Tracking can help improve your dietary habits and achieve your health and wellness goals.

To track your food correctly, you need a way of tracking that works for you.

You can use an app. There are several excellent options out there. Find the one that gives you the information you need. I like the Lose It app. It does much of the work, like calories and macros, and connects to my watch.

You can also buy a food journal. There are so many available out there. If you want to see what you are eating, this works well. If you want to count calories and macros, pen to paper is a bit more work, and we want this to be easier for you.

Portions: this is the key to good tracking. You have to weigh and measure. Remember #1: ½ portions reminds us how important how much we are eating is the key to weight loss. So, learning and tracking portions will help you learn what satisfies you. Buy a good food scale and extra measuring cups and spoons.

Tracking your feelings is a way of recognizing habits and having an outlet to feel your feels.

I have met people who have journaled all their lives. It is part of who they are. I also know this can be very difficult for some of us. If it is hard, it is because we think there is a "right " way. There is not; you do not have to write in complete sentences and paragraphs. You can journal with stick figures and single words; I even have a client who uses emojis and uses colors to express her feelings.

Tracking feelings is an effective tool for improving overall health and wellness.

One of the key benefits of tracking feelings is increased self-awareness. When we track our emotions, we become more mindful of how we feel at any moment and can identify patterns or triggers that may contribute to our emotional state. This self-awareness can help us better understand our emotions and make healthier choices in response to them.

This can also lead to better stress management. When we are more aware of our emotional state, we can identify when we are feeling stressed or overwhelmed and take proactive steps to reduce or manage that stress. This might include practicing relaxation techniques, seeking support from friends or family, or engaging in activities that bring us joy and relaxation.

Another benefit of tracking feelings is improved communication. When we are aware of our own emotions, we can better express them to others clearly and constructively. This can improve our relationships and reduce conflicts by better communicating our needs and boundaries. We will be visiting boundaries soon. This is such an important part of a healthy lifestyle.

Finally, tracking feelings can lead to better overall health and wellness. By identifying and managing negative emotions, we may experience improved mood, better sleep, and reduced physical symptoms such as headaches or stomach aches. This can contribute to an overall sense of well-being and improved quality of life.

I love a beautiful journal and have found that words work for me. They do not have to be just what I am feeling in a sentence. Making time to journal for 5 to 10 minutes daily will help you manage emotions much better. Morning to set intentions for your day. Evening to button up your day.

What App will you use to track? Is it time to buy a new journal?

Use the Always On Your Side Power of 13 Workbook
to personalize your plan.

30.

Chapter 6

Power of 13

#5 Double your Vegetable Intake

~Strive to eat the Rainbow every day~
~Coach Paris~

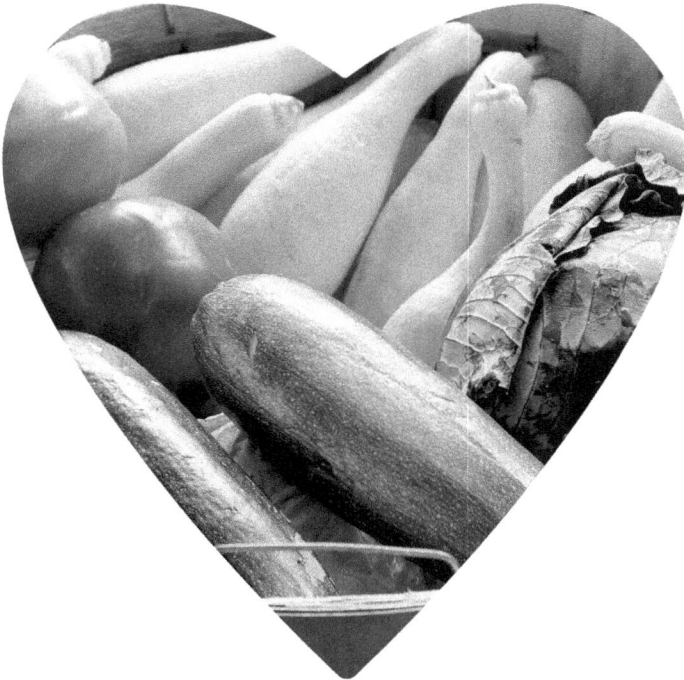

Most of us have a love-hate relationship with vegetables. We know we should eat them, but it is really easy to just skip them. They are not something we necessarily crave, like sweets. Vegetables are important to your health but also help fill you up, so you eat less calorie-laden foods. But double, really? Yes, double. Now for some of you, that will be one serving because you weren't eating before reading this book. For some of you who are really good at getting your vegetables in, doubling may be more than you need. So here is what we are looking for: Work your way up to 5 to 9 half-cup servings (leafy greens are 1 cup) daily. Start slow; your digestive system needs time to adjust. Your goal is to get vegetables every day for most meals and snacks.

The importance of vegetables.

Doubling your vegetable intake can be a highly effective strategy for losing weight. Vegetables are low in calories and high in fiber, which means they can help you feel fuller for extended periods of time while consuming fewer calories overall. Additionally, they are rich in vitamins, minerals, and other important nutrients that can support a healthy metabolism and weight loss.

In addition to being low in calories, vegetables are also high in fiber. Fiber is a carbohydrate that cannot be digested by the body, which means it passes through the digestive system without adding calories. However, it does help slow down the digestion of other foods in the meal, which can help keep you feeling full for extended periods. This can help to reduce overall caloric intake by reducing the likelihood of snacking or overeating later in the day.

Another benefit of vegetables for weight loss is their high nutrient content. Vegetables are rich in vitamins, minerals, and other important nutrients, supporting a healthy metabolism and weight loss. For example, some studies have found that specific vitamins and minerals, such as vitamin C and magnesium, may be associated with lower body weight or BMI.

To double your vegetable intake, consider adding more vegetables to your meals and snacks throughout the day. You can add vegetables to your breakfast by adding spinach to your eggs or making a vegetable-packed smoothie. For lunch and dinner, consider making a salad or vegetable-based soup as a main course or adding more vegetables to your meals. You can also snack on vegetables throughout the day, such as carrot sticks, bell pepper slices, or cherry tomatoes. A positive attitude towards vegetables can also help you get more in.

Challenging the excuses:

Vegetables are expensive. They certainly can be. I suggest buying in season and in sales. Check out the list below. Buying frozen vegetables, the freezer section can be your best friend when something is out of season. Frozen vegetables are frozen at peak season, and you get the best of the best. Stock up or buy fresh and freeze your own. Summer shop farmers markets.

They are too much work. We have all gone to the store, stocked up on all the produce, brought it home, and thought, what have I done? This will all go to waste. I am a prepper who brings everything home and washes, peels, preps, and chops. But that is only realistic for some. I suggest to my clients to buy it prepped. Buy that vegetable tray. It may cost a little more but will get eaten and less waste. The best part is if you find it is getting to the end of its life, you can throw most of it in the freezer to add to soup, stews, or roasts later—so much less waste. Everything freezes except cucumbers. If I have leftover carrots and celery, I chop them small and freeze them as mirepoix.

I don't like vegetables. I hear you, but when did you last try something new? Most of us disliked vegetables when we were little because of the way they were prepped, and we didn't know any better. Boiled vegetables Ugh. Try a new vegetable a week. I suggest that all of my clients roast or air fry their vegetables. They are wonderful. You don't have to love all vegetables;

variety is important, so you continue to eat them and don't get bored, but if you have a good core group of 5 to 7, learn to make them in different ways and enjoy!

Lastly, do not add rich sauces, cheeses, and butter to make them better. This does take away your health benefits. Use olive oil and herbs, and spices to enhance the flavor.

Let's talk about What is in Season.

January: broccoli, brussels sprouts, cauliflower, apples, grapefruit, lemons, navel oranges, papaya, tangerines, tangelos.

February: broccoli, brussels sprouts, cauliflower, apples, oranges, grapefruits, Lemons, papayas.

March: broccoli, mangoes, pineapples.

April: artichokes, asparagus, broccoli, cauliflower, cucumber, rhubarb, spring peas, zucchini, apricots, cherries, mangoes, pineapples, strawberries.

May: artichokes, asparagus, broccoli, cauliflower, cucumber, okra, peppers, rhubarb, spring peas, summer squash, zucchini, apricots, blueberries, cherries, mangoes, pineapples, plums, strawberries.

June: asparagus, beans, cauliflower, corn, cucumber, eggplants, okra, peppers, summer squash, apricots, blueberries, cantaloupe, cherries, mangoes, peaches, plums, strawberries, watermelon.

July: asparagus, beans, cauliflower, corn, cucumber, eggplants, okra, peas, peppers, summer squash, tomatoes, apricots, blackberries, blueberries, cantaloupe, kiwi, peaches, plums, raspberries, strawberries, watermelon.

August: beans, cauliflower, corn, cucumber, eggplant, lettuce, okra, peas, peppers, summer squash, tomatoes, apples, apricots, blackberries, blueberries, cantaloupe, figs, grapes, kiwi, peaches, plums, raspberries, strawberry, watermelon.

September: beans, cauliflower, cucumbers, eggplants, peppers, pumpkin, summer squash, tomatillos, tomatoes, winter squash, apples, figs, grapes, pomegranates, raspberries.

October: broccoli, cauliflower, cucumber, peppers, pumpkins, tomatillos, winter squash, apples, cranberries, grapes, persimmons, pomegranates.

November: broccoli, brussels sprouts, cauliflower, parsnips, pumpkin, winter squash, apples, cranberries, oranges, pears, persimmons, pomegranates, tangerines.

December: broccoli, brussels sprouts, cauliflower, winter squash, apples, grapefruit, oranges, papayas, pears, persimmons, pomegranates, tangerines.

Always in Season: Bananas, beets, cabbage, carrots, lettuce, leeks, mushrooms, onions, parsnips, potatoes, spinach.

Use the Always On Your Side Power of 13 Workbook
to personalize your plan.

Chapter 7

Power of 13

#6 Stretch "on purpose" 10-15 minutes per day

~Stretching Exercises Promote Flexibility, so you move fluidly. ~
~Denise Austin~

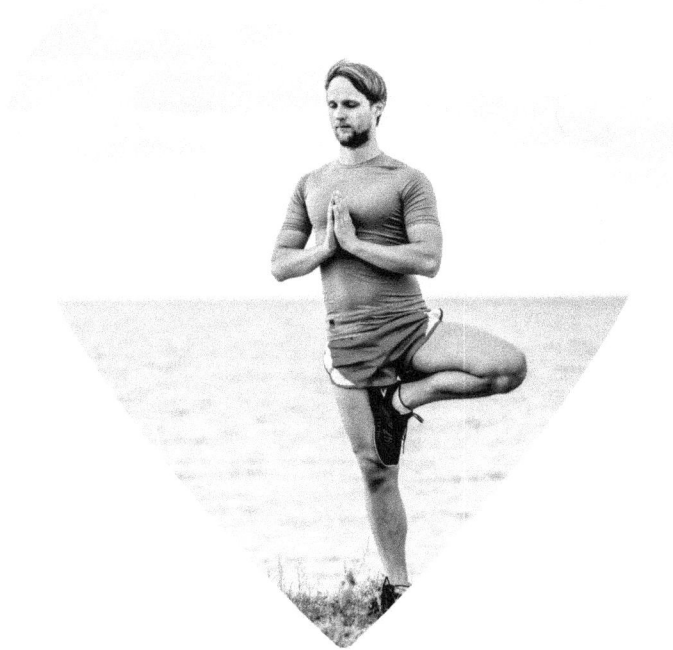

Unfortunately, the older we get, the more we hurt, and the reason for that is that we just don't stretch enough. We don't stretch enough because it hurts to stretch. But we have to. As we age, we need to maintain balance and flexibility to remain independent. I encourage all of my clients to get on the floor several times a day and get back up. Why? Because it builds your strength, your core, and confidence. Some of you say I can't get up once I am there. When you start, be sure you are near a chair or have someone to help, but keep doing it and you will get stronger. It does not matter how you look doing it; just do it. Gracefulness is not required. Here's my promise. You will hurt less the more you stretch. So let's get started.

Stretching Facts:

Improves Flexibility: Stretching is an effective way to improve flexibility and range of motion. Regular stretching can help to lengthen tight muscles and improve joint mobility. This can lead to improved performance in physical activities, such as sports or exercise, and reduce the risk of injury.

Reduces Muscle Tension: Stretching can also help to reduce muscle tension and soreness. When muscles are tight or overused, they can become tense and painful. Stretching can help to release this tension and increase blood flow to the muscles, which can help to reduce soreness and improve recovery after exercise.

Improves Posture: Poor posture is a common problem that can lead to back pain, neck pain, and other health issues. Regular stretching can help to improve posture by lengthening tight muscles and reducing muscle imbalances. This can help to reduce pain and discomfort and improve overall quality of life.

Reduces Stress: Stretching can also be a great way to reduce stress and promote relaxation. When we are stressed, our muscles can become tense and tight. Stretching can help release this tension and promote calm and relaxation.

Promotes Circulation: Stretching can also help to promote circulation throughout the body. When we stretch, blood flow to the muscles increases, which can help deliver oxygen and nutrients to the muscles and improve overall health and well-being.

Incorporating stretching into your daily routine can be a simple and effective way to improve your overall quality of life.

How to get started.

One of my favorite things about stretching is that I don't have to jump out of bed to do it. Start 1st thing in the morning while you are still in bed. Full body morning stretch. Head side to side. Shoulders to ears. Knees to chest. Whatever helps you wake up.

Stretch while doing other activities, cooking, brushing your teeth, showering, or on a call.

Before bed, some slow, steady stretching at the end of your day can calm your body and help you sleep better and wake less because of pain.

One last little fun thing. My family had greyhounds, and those pups knew how to stretch often and deep. Suppose you have a dog or cat. They stretch all the time; watch them. Every time your pet stretches, you stretch!

Use the Always On Your Side Power of 13 Workbook
to personalize your plan.

Power of 13

#7 Read something positive each day for at least 15 minutes a day

~Use reading to lift you up and encourage you each day. ~
~Coach Paris

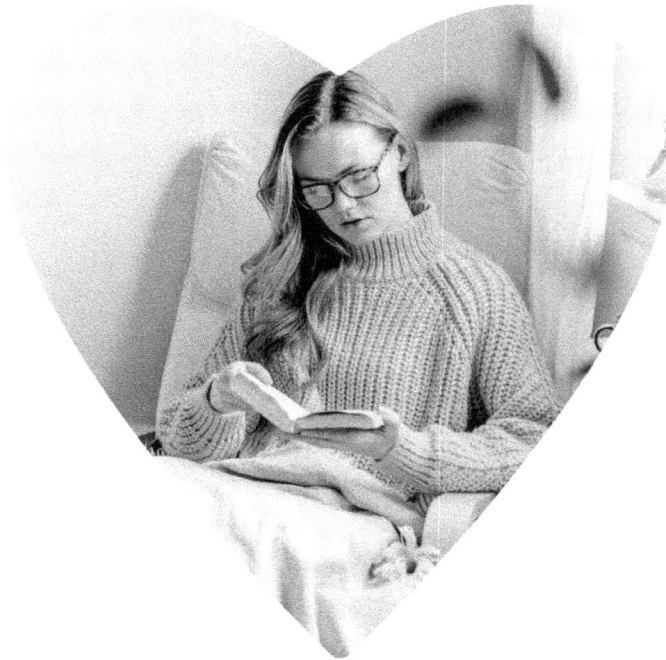

We are bombarded with information and negativity every single day. We have access to so much information we can look anything up in a split second, and we believe it must be true if it is on the internet. We seldom take time to look for positive stories or information. It never tops our feed on our social media. Reading something positive is important because it can significantly impact our mental and emotional well-being. Positive reading material, such as uplifting stories, inspiring quotes, or self-help books, can help to boost our mood, reduce stress and anxiety, and increase our sense of optimism and hope. Reading Keeps Your Brain Healthy and Helps You Sleep Better. It can also improve our perspective and outlook on life, allowing us to focus on the good in the world and cultivate a more positive attitude towards ourselves and others. Reading positive material can also provide us with a sense of motivation and inspiration, encouraging us to pursue our goals and dreams with renewed vigor and enthusiasm. Reading something positive can effectively promote happiness, resilience, and personal growth in our lives.

Read comics, self-help books, positive affirmations, and devotionals. I love daily affirmation books. I also love reading other people's success stories. Find what lifts you and create a 15-minute habit.

What will you read today?

Use the Always On Your Side Power of 13 Workbook
to personalize your plan.

42.

Chapter 9

Power of 13

#8 Learn about and Incorporate healthy fats each day

~A perfectly working body requires Healthy fats.~
~Coach Paris~

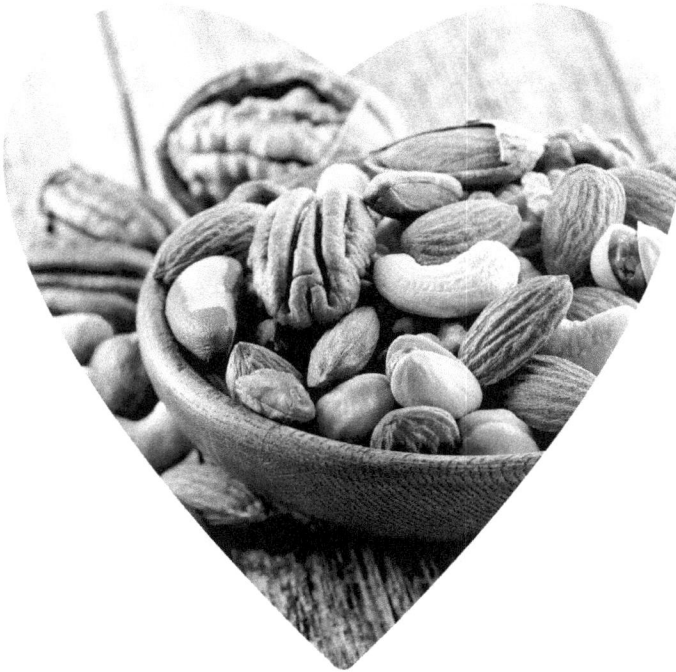

Fat-free diets were so popular in the '70s. They convinced us that all fat was bad. We cut it all out and believed everything we heard. Then our hair started falling out, we lost muscle mass, and our skin and nails were flaking off. We were losing focus and concentration. Plus, we were starving and eating more junk. Fast forward to now, and we know we need healthy fats in our daily diet. When most people think of losing weight, they often think of cutting out fats from their diet. However, not all fats are created equal. Consuming the right kinds of fats can assist in weight loss. There is also a lot of information out there that is terribly confusing. We hear coconut oil and butter are OK fat sources in your daily diet. I will tell you NO; they are loaded with saturated fat and will negatively impact your health no matter how you look at it. Ask any cardiologist.

Why and how much do we need?

Healthy fats can help you feel full: Foods that contain healthy fats, such as nuts, avocados, and olive oil, are often high in fiber and protein, which can help you feel fuller for longer periods of time. This can lead to consuming fewer calories throughout the day, making it easier to stay in a calorie deficit necessary for weight loss.

They can boost metabolism: Some studies have shown that consuming healthy fats can boost metabolism, which can help to burn more calories throughout the day. This is because healthy fats can stimulate the production of hormones that help to regulate metabolism and increase fat burning.

They reduce inflammation: Chronic inflammation has been linked to obesity and other health problems. Healthy fats, such as those found in fish and nuts, contain anti-inflammatory properties that can help to reduce inflammation in the body. This can improve health and aid in weight loss.

They improve nutrient absorption: Vitamins A, D, E, and K are all fat-soluble, which means they need fat to be properly absorbed and utilized by the body. Consuming healthy fats can help the body absorb these essential nutrients.

Healthy fats can improve insulin sensitivity: Insulin is a hormone that regulates blood sugar levels in the body. Consuming healthy fats can help to improve insulin sensitivity, which can help to prevent insulin resistance and type 2 diabetes, both of which are associated with weight gain.

Suggested amounts

Total fat: 20% to 35% of daily calories
Saturated fat: 10% or less of daily calories

Let's break them down.

The worst type of dietary fat is the kind known as trans fat.
Trans fats have no known health benefits, and there is no safe level of consumption. Therefore, they have been officially banned in the United States.

Saturated fats are common in the American diet. These are Bad fats.

They are solid at room temperature — think cooled bacon grease, but what is saturated fat? Saturated fat includes red meat, whole milk, and other whole-milk dairy foods, cheese, coconut oil, and many commercially prepared baked goods and other foods.

Is saturated fat bad for you? A diet rich in saturated fats can drive up total cholesterol and tip the balance toward more harmful LDL cholesterol, prompting blockages in arteries in the heart and elsewhere in the body. Therefore, we are recommended to limit saturated fat to under 10% of calories a day.

Good fats come mainly from vegetables, nuts, seeds, and fish.

They differ from saturated fats by having fewer hydrogen atoms bonded to their carbon chains. Healthy fats are liquid at room temperature, not solid. There are two broad categories of beneficial fats: monounsaturated and polyunsaturated fats.

Best sources of Good fats that do not cause inflammation:

The only two oils you need in your kitchen
Extra virgin olive oil: is great for dipping, finishing foods, and homemade salad dressings. You can cook with it at lower temperatures.
Avocado oil: has a high smoke point, so it is great for roasting and frying.
Fatty fish, including wild-caught salmon, are best, as mackerel, cod, trout, sardines, haddock, and tuna.
Avocados and olives
Nuts and nut butters (natural check ingredients should only have nuts and salt.)

A few ways to add healthy fats every day:

Eat more fish
Cook your eggs in avocado or olive oil instead of spray. While the spray may save calories, the healthy fat will keep you full longer.
Avocado or nut butter toast
Add nuts to your yogurt or oatmeal
Make homemade salad dressings with olive oil, vinegars, and spices
Stuff celery with nut butters

46.

Nut butter sandwiches
Cook chicken breasts or other lean proteins in olive or avocado oil
Hummus or guacamole and vegetables
Nut butter and apples
Use olive or avocado oil in your sauces and cooking proteins
Add nuts or avocado to salads
Use olives in your cooking, add to salads, Mexican entrees, and even pizza
Portion our nuts for snacks

To monitor the fat in your diet, add the fat grams from the foods you ate during the day. Use the Nutrition Facts label to determine how much fat is in your foods.

Remembering it is important to get the healthy fats in your diet, here's what you will notice if you get enough.

Feeling full
Healthy skin, hair, and nails
Better concentration and focus
The digestive system will work correctly

It is important to note that while healthy fats can aid in weight loss, they should be consumed in moderation as they are still high in calories. The key is to focus on incorporating healthy fats into a balanced and nutritious diet rather than solely relying on them for weight loss. Portion control matters. Use your measuring spoons.

Use the Always On Your Side Power of 13 Workbook
to personalize your plan.

Power of 13

#9 Eat fruit, portion-controlled, each day

The Perfect way to add to your rainbow each day.
~Coach Paris

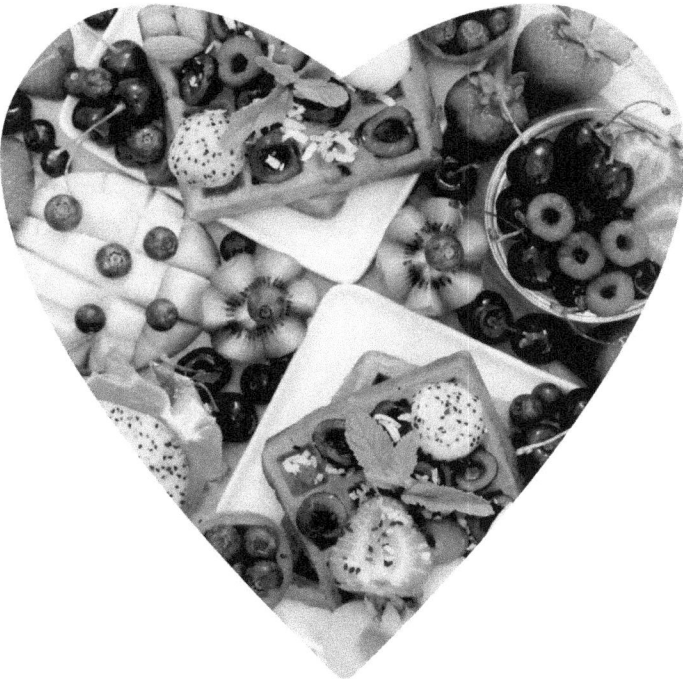

Like vegetables, we should incorporate fruits into our daily diet. It is also easier for most people to get the fruits every day. However, your fruit intake must be portion controlled and limited. Why? Fruit is very important in a healthy diet; giving us important nutrients and choosing it over high sugar and fat options will help with weight loss. But it is also something that needs to be limited. Fruit varies highly in calories and some are quite high. Calories matter no matter what it is we are eating. The argument can be made, but it has to be better if I have grapes instead of M&M's. You are right, but a pound of grapes (306) and a small bag of M&Ms (230) may have nearly the same calories. Choose the grapes every single time but portion controlled. A lady once told me she ate a whole watermelon in a day. That's a lot of watermelon and a lot of calories. Some fruits are higher in sugar, and while naturally occurring sugar is digested slower and helps you feel full for longer, calories still matter.

Fruit is a crucial component of a healthy and balanced diet, and incorporating it into your daily routine can have numerous benefits for your health and wellness journey.

They are an excellent source of essential vitamins and minerals for optimal health. For example, citrus fruits such as oranges and grapefruits are rich in vitamin C, which is key in supporting the immune system and promoting healthy skin. Similarly, berries are packed with antioxidants, which can help to protect your cells from damage and reduce your risk of chronic diseases.

In addition to providing essential nutrients, they are also a great source of dietary fiber, which plays an important role in digestive health by helping to regulate bowel movements and prevent constipation. It can also help promote feelings of fullness, which can benefit weight management.

Another benefit of fruit is that it can help to reduce the risk of chronic diseases such as heart disease, stroke, and diabetes. This is because it is low in fat and calories and high in nutrients.

Furthermore, incorporating fruit into your diet can be a great way to satisfy your sweet tooth without relying on processed or sugary foods. It is a natural source of sweetness and can be used in various ways to create delicious and healthy snacks and desserts.

Best fruits overall:
Berries: Blueberries, strawberries, blackberries and raspberries, and boysenberries.
Fruits with the least amount of Sugar (Low glycemic)
Cherries, grapefruit, dried apricots, pears, apples, oranges, plums, strawberries.
Fruits with the Highest amount of sugar (High glycemic)
Bananas, oranges, mango, grapes, raisins, dates, and pears.

Use the Always On Your Side Power of 13 Workbook
to personalize your plan.

Power of 13

#10 Create boundaries and enforce them

~ Setting boundaries is a form of self-respect.~
~Coach Paris

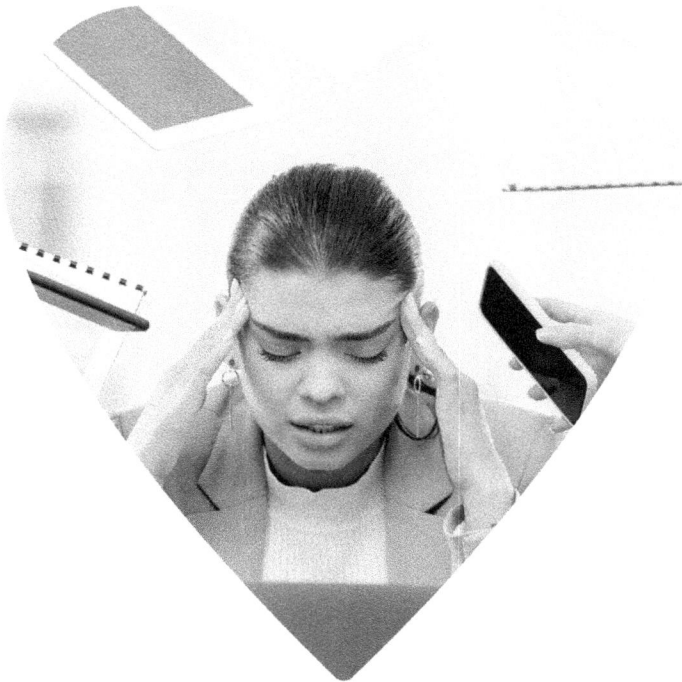

Covid was the beginning for me as a coach seeing how quickly people let go of boundaries. When we all started working from home, we lost our work boundaries. We started working longer hours with no "quitting" time; we no longer closed the door and drove home. We answered emails late into the night; we became less efficient in our work days because we could work later. We gave up our free time because there was nothing to do anyway.

Then when everything opened back up, we couldn't say No to anything. We did not want to miss out on anything. Fear of missing out (FOMO) So we overbooked and over-extended. Then we started to complain about being tired and worn out. We kept saying yes for fear of letting someone down or hurting someone's feelings."No is a complete sentence" is some of the best advice I have received.

Regarding boundaries with family, children, spouses, or even parents:

Teaching others how to do things for themselves is where you start to set boundaries and realize you do not need to control everything. Let go and remember your way may only sometimes be the right way. Personal Boundaries are important because they set the basic guidelines of how you want to be treated.

We need boundaries in all areas of our lives.

Boundaries are essential to maintaining healthy relationships and protecting our mental and emotional well-being. They allow us to define acceptable behavior and not communicate our needs and expectations to others.

They help us establish a sense of personal identity and self-worth. We communicate to others that we have a sense of self-respect and that our needs and feelings are valid. This can help us build self-confidence and a positive self-image.

54.

They help us maintain healthy relationships by defining acceptable behavior and what is not. For example, if we establish boundaries around communication, we can let others know what types of conversations are acceptable and what types are not. This can help to prevent misunderstandings and conflicts in our relationships.

In addition, it can help to protect our mental and emotional well-being by allowing us to control our exposure to stress and negativity. When we establish boundaries around our time, energy, and emotional availability, we can prevent others from taking advantage of or draining us emotionally. This can help us to maintain a healthy balance in our lives and to avoid burnout or exhaustion.

Boundaries can also help us to manage our behavior and emotions. By establishing limits around our actions and thoughts, we can prevent ourselves from engaging in harmful or self-destructive behaviors and cultivate greater self-awareness and self-control.

Who in your life these days do you need to set boundaries with? Recognizing and communicating what you need is how we start setting the boundaries we need.

Use the Always On Your Side Power of 13 Workbook
to personalize your plan.

Chapter 12

Power of 13

#11 Weight-bearing activity - 15 to 30 minutes per day, 2 days a week

~Muscle makes everything feel, look and work better ~
~Coach Paris

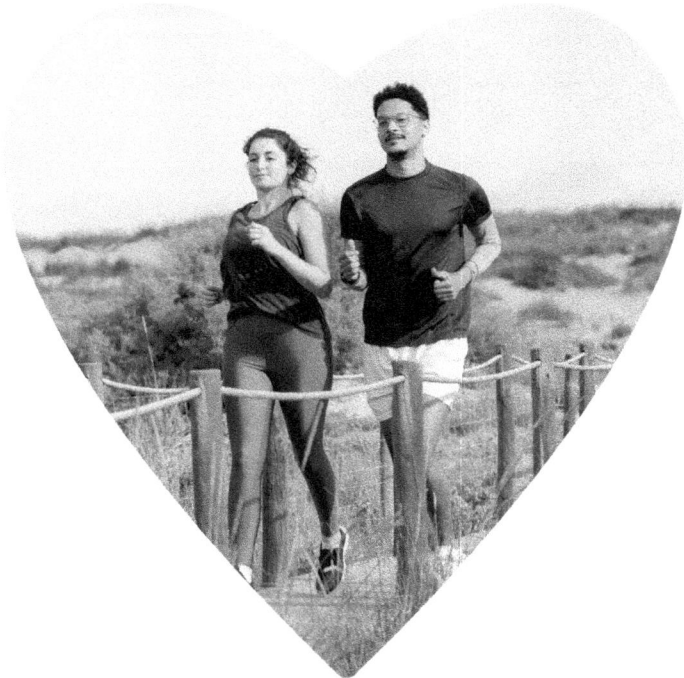

I always thought I had to go to the gym and do the heavy lifting to be considered a weight-bearing activity. I also always loved hearing people say I don't want to be muscle-bound. All of those things could not be further from the truth regarding weight-bearing activity. I learned about it in my health and nutrition courses and knew it had to be part of the Power of 13.

Weight-bearing activities involve supporting your own body weight through your feet and legs. This type of activity is essential for maintaining bone health, improving balance and coordination, and promoting overall fitness and well-being.

They require your bones to bear your body's weight, which helps stimulate bone growth and strengthen your skeletal system. This can be especially important for older adults, as age-related bone loss can increase the risk of osteoporosis and fractures.

In addition to promoting bone health, they also offer a number of other benefits. They can help to improve cardiovascular health by increasing heart rate and improving circulation. They can also help to build muscle mass and improve overall strength and endurance.

These activities can also be an effective way to manage weight and prevent obesity. They burn calories and can help to build lean muscle mass, which can help to boost metabolism and promote healthy weight loss.

They can also be a great way to improve balance and coordination. This can be especially important for older adults, as falls are a leading cause of injury and disability in this population. By improving balance and coordination, weight-bearing activities can help to prevent falls and improve overall mobility.

58.

What is considered a weight-bearing activity? You may already be doing some of these things as your 30 minutes a day.

Walking, running, jumping rope, dancing, aerobics, hiking, elliptical machines, stair climbing, and weightlifting.

Let's lace up our shoes and get moving!

Use the Always On Your Side Power of 13 Workbook
to personalize your plan.

Power of 13

#12 Limit White foods, Sugar, Salt, Flour, Rice, and Pasta.

~There is not one health benefit to white foods.
Reduce your intake and feel better fast~
~Coach Paris~

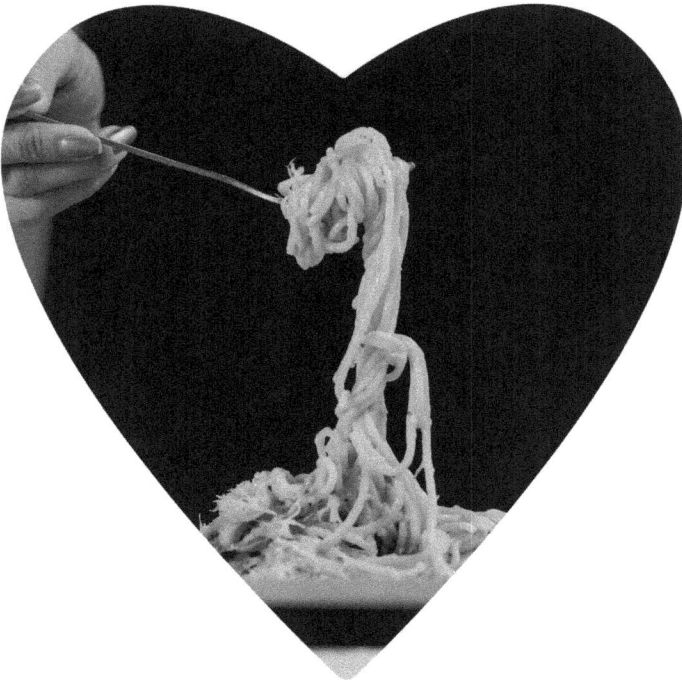

They are our favorites. They taste good, they are usually convenient, and we crave these foods. White food generally refers to foods that have been processed and refined. They often cause overeating, hunger, and cravings. They have no health benefits.

White foods such as sugar, salt, flour, rice, and bread are often heavily processed and refined, stripping away important nutrients and fiber. This means that they are often high in calories and low in nutritional value, making them less healthy than whole foods.

Here are some reasons why we need to limit our consumption of these white foods:

High in sugar: Foods such as sugar and white bread are high in added sugars. Consuming too much sugar can lead to health problems like weight gain, type 2 diabetes, and cardiovascular disease.

High in salt: Processed foods like white bread and packaged snacks often contain high sodium levels. Too much salt can increase blood pressure, leading to heart disease, stroke, and other health issues.

Low in fiber: Refined grains like white rice and flour have had their fiber stripped away, which can cause blood sugar spikes and leave you feeling hungry soon after eating. Fiber is important for digestion, weight management, and overall health.

Can contribute to overeating: These foods are often high in calories and low in nutritional value, which can lead to overeating and weight gain. In contrast, whole foods like fruits, vegetables, and whole grains are nutrient-dense and can help you feel full and satisfied.

Lack of nutrients: They lack important vitamins and minerals, such as B vitamins, iron, and fiber. This means consuming too many of them can lead to nutrient deficiencies, negatively impacting your health.

But how do we start to limit these foods? You must let go of your limiting beliefs and try new things. We have all had a bad experience with whole grain pasta or long grain rice. Sticky, pasty, gummy pasta is not very appetizing. They have come a long way over the years, and if it has been a long time since you tried them, try again. Follow the package directions closely. When I cook whole wheat pastas, I cook exactly as it says in the package directions and run under cold water to stop the cooking process, then add to a hot saucepan.

Words on labels that matter when finding breads, crackers, and snacks. Look at your ingredient list and avoid enriched and fortified. Look for Whole wheat or grain as the 1st ingredient.

Try some of these grains to replace white rice snacks and pastas.

Barley, Bulgur, also called cracked wheat, farro, millet, quinoa, black rice, brown rice, red rice, wild rice, oatmeal, popcorn, and whole-wheat flour. Whole-grain breakfast cereals and whole-wheat bread, pasta, or crackers.

Sugar: Natural Occurring vs. Added

Natural sugars are found in fruit as fructose and in dairy products, such as milk and cheese, as lactose. These foods contain essential nutrients that keep the body healthy and help prevent disease. Natural sources of sugar are digested slower and help you feel full for longer. It also helps keep your metabolism stable.

Refined sugar, or sucrose, comes from sugar cane or sugar beets, which are processed to extract the sugar. Food manufacturers add chemically produced sugar, typically high-fructose corn syrup, to many packaged foods. The body breaks down refined sugar rapidly, which causes insulin and blood sugar levels to skyrocket. Since it is digested quickly, you don't feel full after eating, regardless of how much you ate. Increased consumption of refined sugar has been linked to the rise in obesity rates, which is associated with higher cancer risks.

All forms of added sugar have no nutritional benefit at all. No one sugar is better than another. Brown sugar, corn sweetener, corn syrup, fruit juice concentrates, high-fructose corn syrup, honey, inverted sugar, malt sugar, molasses, raw sugar (turbinado), sugar, sugar molecules (dextrose, fructose, glucose, lactose, maltose, sucrose), syrup, they are all equally bad. You would quickly notice how much better you felt if you gave them up completely. But giving up added sugar completely takes work. It is in everything. Added sugars are now on all nutrition labels, so we can educate ourselves by looking at those before purchasing packaged foods. A good rule of thumb is to leave it with more than two grams of sugar. Several places to look closely are yogurts (there will be sugar in yogurt but look closely at the added), cereals, breads, protein bars, and shakes.

How Much?

We should limit our added sugar to no more than 25 grams daily, six teaspoons, or 100 calories. One 12 oz Coke has seven teaspoons.

Like Sugar: Sodium is in everything. But our bodies do need salt. But we don't need to have it at the dining table. It is hard to avoid salt completely, so you probably get plenty in your daily diet. Too much sodium is the leading cause of high blood pressure, which leads to strokes and heart disease. Limit your sodium each day to below 1500 MG.

64.

Educate yourself and eat less processed food to lower your white food intake.

Use the Always On Your Side Power
of 13 Workbook to personalize your plan.

Chapter 14

Power of 13

#13 Pause and be mindful every day

~Pausing before anything goes in or comes out of your mouth will always
have a positive outcome~
~Coach Paris

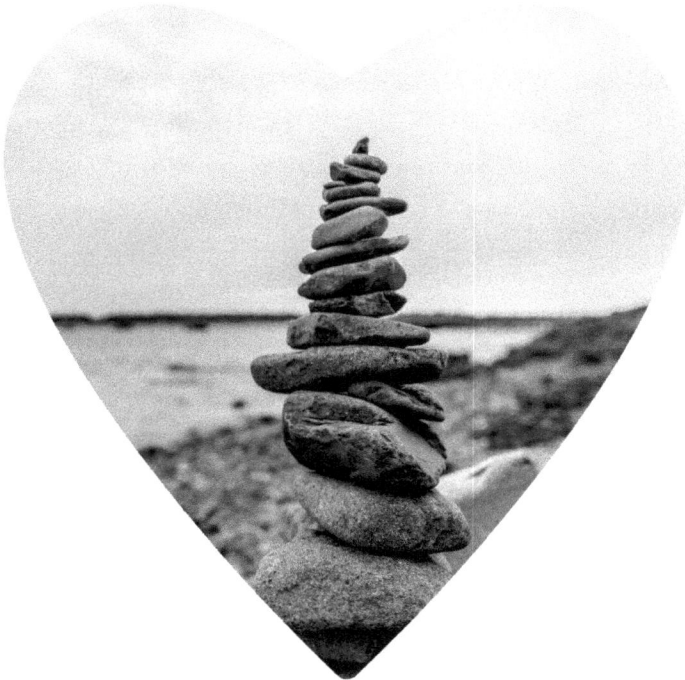

Pausing is a form of self-control. There is a positive outcome when we practice "the pause" 85% of the time. Pause before you react, before you grab a snack, before you speak, and even before you make small decisions. We will make better choices if we pause before we open our mouths, whether to speak or eat.

Here are some reasons why it is important to pause:

Rest and recharge: Taking breaks from our work or daily routines allows us to rest and recharge our batteries. This can help us feel more energized, focused, and productive when we return to our tasks.

Reduce stress: Pausing and taking a break can help reduce stress levels by allowing our minds and bodies to relax and unwind. This can also help us gain perspective and approach our challenges with a clearer, more positive mindset.

Improve decision-making: When we're constantly on the go, making thoughtful and informed decisions can be challenging. Taking time to reflect can help us make better decisions by allowing us to weigh our options and consider the consequences of our choices.

Increase creativity: Pausing can also increase creativity by allowing our minds to wander and explore new ideas. A break from our routine can help us see things from a different perspective and come up with fresh solutions to our problems.

Connect with ourselves and others: Finally, pausing can help us connect with ourselves and others. By reflecting on our experiences and emotions, we can better understand ourselves and our relationships with those around us.

68.

You should have a question to ask yourself in these situations.

Start with the technique Pause 5~4~3~2~1. Breathe and ask

Before you grab a snack or eat a meal:

- Will this get me closer to my goal?
- How will I feel after I eat this?
- Is this my best choice?

Before you offer advice or tell your experience:

- Did they ask for my advice?
- Will my story help?
- Is what I have to say important or warranted?

Before you react:

- What do I control in this situation?
- Am I reacting with the correct person?
- Will my feelings make a difference?

Sometimes it is just better to pause to learn more about yourself.

Use the Always On Your Side Power
of 13 Workbook to personalize your plan.

Chapter 15

A few more things worth mentioning

"There is always more to learn."
~Coach Paris

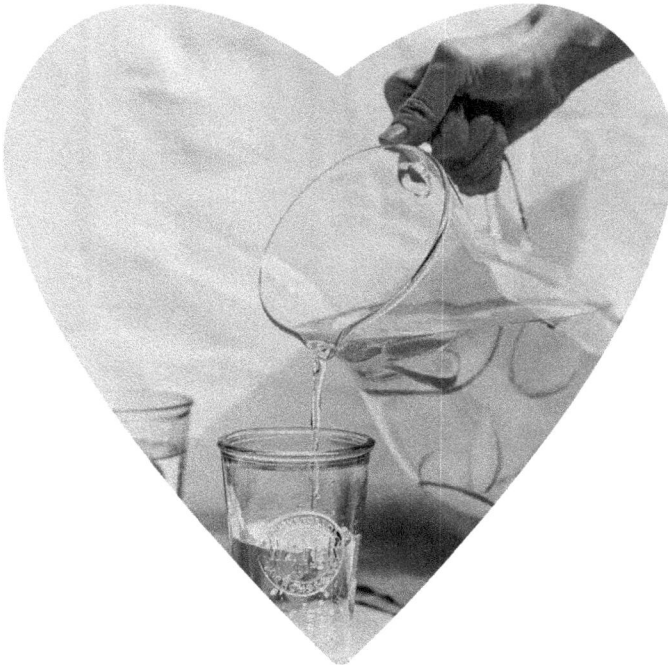

Water: why we need it.

Healthy heart, more energy, decreased joint pain, temperature regulation.

Digestive regularity and kidney stone prevention.

Weight loss and management: water helps you feel full. Drink 8 oz before each meal.

Brain: even just being 2% dehydrated can cause you to affect reaction times, memory, focus, and concentration.

How much do we need? The answer is all over the place, from 24 ounces to ½ your body weight to 100 ounces. Getting 48 to 64 ounces of plain water every single day will keep most of us hydrated but listen to your body. If you are thirsty, drink more.

How to get it? This is a personal preference. I always use a straw and drink much more water when it is not ice cold. Winter is a struggle for me because I hate getting cold. I recently started drinking hot water to warm up and found myself drinking 64 oz daily with no problem. I also found I don't like water bottles more than 24 oz. I never seem to finish them, but my 18 oz I fill up several times a day. I have a client with a 64 oz cup that works great for her. Try different things to find how getting your water finished each day is easier.

Vitamins and Supplements:

This is a hot button for some people, and I will tell you you need only a few different things.

Eating a primarily clean diet requires a good multi-vitamin with 100% RDA of vitamins and minerals. Your vitamins should never be gummies; they are loaded with added sugar you don't need.

A daily probiotic to keep your gut happy and healthy. Our environment has many pollutants, and our foods will help protect our immune and digestive systems.

Muscle does NOT weigh more than fat.

No matter what you have read, muscle does not weigh more than fat. A pound is a pound. Muscle does take up less space. You will look better in (and out) of your clothes. The other benefit of more muscle is a better working metabolism. The more muscle you have the faster you will burn calories.

You can't outrun your fork.

Weight loss is 80% what you eat and 20% activity. It takes a lot of exercise to burn calories. The best example I have ever heard is to burn one plain M&M, you have to walk the length of a football field. Wow, one bag is a lot of football fields. When you are losing weight, you have to change your diet. Using activity for everything else in your life: stress relief, tightening up your body as you lose, feel-good endorphins, and managing your mindset. To see the number on the scale change, eat smaller portions, less saturated fat, and added sugar. Don't count on activity to get you to your weight loss goals.

I hope that this gives you easy-to-follow directions to a healthy lifestyle. Weight loss and maintenance are something you never get to quit. You need to incorporate the Power of 13 for the rest of your life. But knowing you have these tools will make it manageable.

Never ever give up. If you stumble, it's ok; just begin again. A healthy lifestyle is a slippery slope. You will not always be perfect and you don't have to be, to be successful. It's very forgiving.

Be sure to sign up for updates on our website. Alwaysonyoursidecoaching. com

Learn more about our Offerings there too.

We have Virtual 1:1 Coaching and Weekly Support groups available.

Coming 2024:

We will have both online and in-person 12-week Always On Your Side Power of 13 Coaching courses.

Here's to your best health,
~Coach Paris

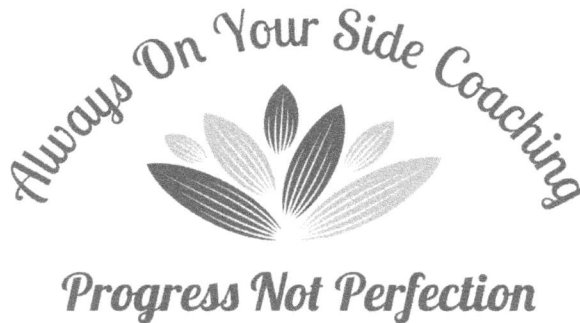

Always On Your Side Coaching

Progress Not Perfection

74.

Chapter 16

What people are saying

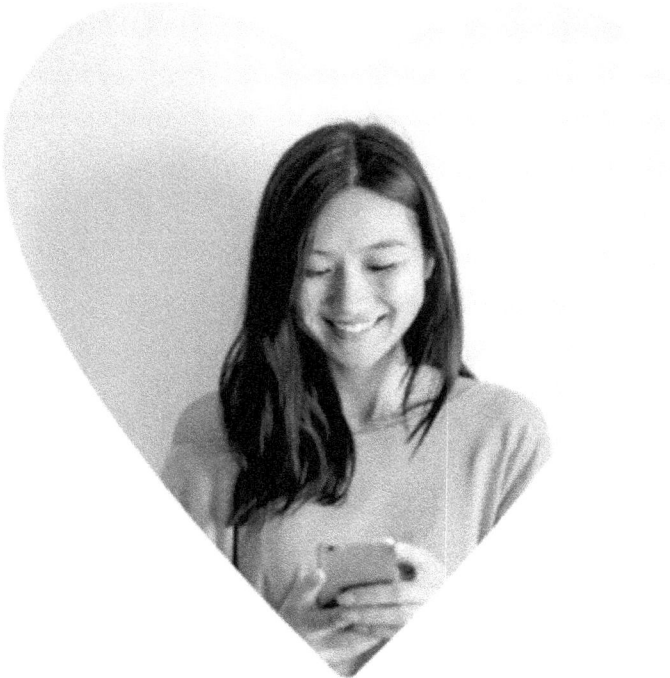

AOYS Power of 13 has been helping Clients in support groups and one-on-one coaching since 2021. Here is what our clients are saying:

The Power of 13 are ideas to live by and have become integral in my life now and know if I am even hitting a few of them daily, I am successful at working towards a long and healthy life. There are different approaches to all of them, and as long as you put effort into balancing them, they are easy to live by. **~Deb A**

Ways you have helped me...
- not just focused on weight loss, you're a Life Coach (this set you apart in WW too)
- built a community that provides a support group
- flexible in meeting people where they're at, no judgment
- not a one size fits all approach
- Power of 13 is practical and do-able, especially because you're so clear that it's not 100% of them 100% of the time
- you do research and get certified in a variety of areas so you can talk from a deeper, more real perspective than just a predetermined script. **~Jill R**

Eat half! Work travel was my number 1 healthy eating frustration. Isolated destinations often takeaway healthy options. I ordered the best I could and ate half. This was a game-changer :) **~Laura T**

Paris and the Power of 13 has helped me in countless ways in each category, mostly my portion control, planning, and fitting my exercise in each day. **~G Downer**

76.

I have an incredible relationship with Paris. I remember the first time I met her at a Weight Watcher's meeting about 25 years ago or more. She was subbing for our leader, but I knew she was something special from that very first meeting. I saw her sparkle then, and I continue to see it today in my AOYS Saturday meetings now. She has taught me how to navigate this crazy world through her life coaching, not just weight coaching, but life. Everything about Paris is pure gold and I consider her my teacher and my friend. ~**Pam M.**

Power of 13 has helped me tremendously. It's made me do things (or at least try) that I never thought I could do before and turn those things into good healthy habits. Paris is so inspiring and a wonderful person to have as a coach in all aspects of life. She's my rock. ~**Carol W**

Coach Paris has helped me with her informative, supportive support groups that I always find a way to attend, no matter how busy I am. I love how I have learned from her that eating half is actually enough, but she is in no way judgmental. She says to start there, and you can always add. She lets everyone find their healthy lifestyle and supports it. Power of 13 has helped me with moving, eating half, and prioritizing sleep. LIFE CHANGING. The education she provides is thought-provoking and eye-opening. ~**Darlene B**

Paris created Always On Your Side Coaching and the Power of 13. Both give a new perspective on nutritional information to aid us on the weight loss journey and make us rethink what we thought we knew. This helps keep this journey fresh and focus on our health goals and gives us a guide to assist us. This is just like having Paris in our back pocket anytime we find ourselves with questions along the way (aka - what would Paris do?) ~**Harriett G**

I've been working with Paris for years and am always amazed at her breadth of knowledge. She doesn't focus on just one 'diet' but instead takes a holistic approach to healthy living. I learn something new every time I talk to Paris, and her positive attitude is contagious. From weekly support groups to one-on-one coaching, she is a great resource and a delight to work with. I feel lucky that I found her and that she's truly always on my side. ~**Kimberly H**

I feel she is always around, which makes me accountable. ~**Kathy G**

Always On Your Side Power of 13 has been helpful to us in three ways:
1. It has affirmed the positive effects of things we have already been doing.
2. It has motivated us to work harder on things we had only half-heartedly begun.
3. It has challenged us to incorporate things we hadn't even considered into our routines.

Paris is a very inspiring coach, always pushing us forward with positive encouragement and well-researched information. We look forward to our weekly support group and the great ideas we get from Paris and each other. ~**John and Kathy Kron**

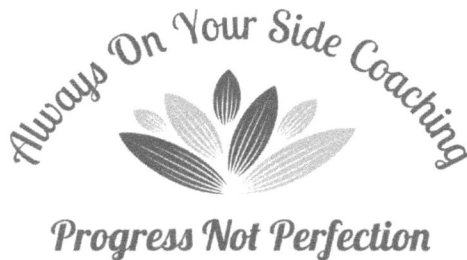

Always On Your Side Coaching

Progress Not Perfection

Chapter 17

Meet Coach Paris

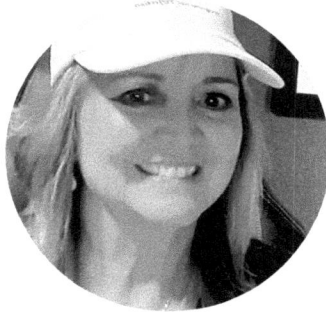

Paris Heinen is a Certified Master Life Coach with certifications in Health and Nutrition, Goal Setting, Life Purpose, Happiness, Self Care, Meditation, and Group Support. With over 23 years of coaching experience, she is an expert in human behavior, helping others realize how their limiting beliefs hold them back. She believes everyone is capable of a healthy lifestyle. She also believes exactly what you want once you stop making excuses.

Her weight loss journey began in 1991; she joined Weight Watchers and lost 55 lbs only to leave the program and regain it. She returned in 2000 and lost 65 lbs. She became a Top Leader for Weight Watchers and worked there for 20 years before leaving and opening her Coaching Practice in January 2021. She created the Power of 13 on a legal pad at her kitchen table. Her coaching practice includes both One on One coaching and Weekly Support Groups.

Paris lives in Highlands Ranch, Colorado, and has been happily married for 35 years to her husband, Don. She has two children and three grandchildren—one bonus daughter with two more grandbabies.

Reference

American Diabetes Association | Research, Education, Advocacy. (n.d.).
https://diabetes.org/

American Heart Association | To be a relentless force for a world of longer, healthier lives. (n.d.). www.heart.org. https://www.heart.org/

New Skills Academy. (n.d.). Online Courses & Qualifications | New Skills Academy. https://newskillsacademy.com/

Rivera, J. &. N. (2023, January 30). *Home - Transformation Academy.* Transformation Academy. https://transformationacademy.com/

WebMD - Better information. Better health. (2023, June 26). WebMD. https://www.webmd.com/WebMD - Better information. Better health. (2023, June 26). WebMD. https://www.webmd.com/

80.

Kindly leave a favorable review

Scan the above QR code
Click on the book link
Skip to #4

1. Log into your Amazon account.
2. Click on Your Account (3 lines)
3. Click on Your Orders: Click on the purchase of this book
4. Scroll to the bottom of the page to Customer Reviews
5. Leave a Favorable Review. ☆☆☆☆☆
   Bonus points for sharing a Video/Photo in the Review.

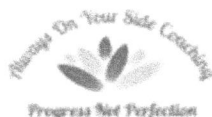

Always On Your Side Coaching
Progress Not Perfection

Thank you!

www.ingramcontent.com/pod-product-compliance
Lightning Source LLC
Chambersburg PA
CBHW052025030426
42335CB00026B/3291